REDUCE MENTAL HEALTH STIGMA IN THE WORKPLACE

5 WAYS TO SAVE MONEY AND SUPPORT YOUR LOCAL COMMUNITY

JEFFY WONG

ISBN: 978-1928155928

PUBLISHED BY:
10-10-10 PUBLISHING
MARKHAM, ON
CANADA

Contents

Foreword

Welcome to a book with the potential to create positive social change around the world. I truly believe that, if it's read by enough of the right people, author Jeffy Wong's message can act as a catalyst for a long-overdue revolution in the way that communities everywhere face the task of helping people who contend with mental health problems to recover and thrive once again. By choosing to read this book, you are demonstrating a desire to move beyond stigma against a group of people who, far from being a burden to society, represent a rich untapped resource that has been left undiscovered for far too long. I wish to thank you first and foremost for the commitment you've shown to changing the status quo, just by picking up this book and reading it.

Jeffy Wong is uniquely poised to lead this revolution, as someone who has himself overcome significant mental health challenges as a result of a brain tumour that was removed early in 1998. Like so many people who are blindsided by mental health problems, it took tremendous courage and determination for Jeffy to overcome the worst of his challenges, but the support he found in the Mosaic Clubhouse community has made it possible for him (and many others) to rebuild the skills, confidence, and self-acceptance they need to lead highly-productive lives. It is his passion for the Clubhouse model of recovery, particularly with regard to its employment initiatives which serve to help people with mental health problems get back to work, that inspired Jeffy to write this book in an effort to spread the word among members of the business community. I know that by the time you've finished reading it, the spark of his passion will have ignited a flame in you as well.

Here is a sampling of what you'll learn within the pages of this enlightening book:

- What stigma against mental ill health looks like, why it is time to transcend it, and how this can be accomplished in our lifetime
- Why Clubhouse International's model of recovery is so effective that it won the world's largest humanitarian cash prize – $4 million US from the Conrad N. Hilton foundation – in 2014.
- How Clubhouse Transitional Employment Programs (TEPs) offer valuable human resource solutions to businesses large and small, even as they create

opportunity for individuals in recovery from mental health problems

This book is not only informative and compelling, it is also an enjoyable read. I hope that you will read it all the way through and let it inspire you to do what you can to remove the barrier of stigma everywhere, but particularly in the workplace. If you are a business owner, you have an invaluable opportunity to, as the Wall Street Journal put it in a recent article about the Clubhouse model, 'do well by doing good.' Nothing feels better than that!

Here's to a new age of empowerment and the end of stigma everywhere.

Raymond Aaron
New York Times Best-selling Author

Testimonial

At a time when the world is just at the edge of meaningful conversation about the need to acknowledge and address the issues of mental illness, Jeffy Wong has written a moving and inspirational book that speaks to the heart of the matter. In an engaging account of his own experience he quickly brings the enormous topic of misunderstanding and prejudice about mental illness to a personal and easy to understand level. From there he artfully leads us on a journey of learning what is possible when there is effective support and reasonable accommodation for individuals on their road to recovery. With Mosaic Clubhouse as an example and the stories of real people and their success, he shows us how government and the business community can both participate and benefit from partnering with a Clubhouse community. This is a book that needs to be read by many.

Joel D. Corcoran
Executive Director
Clubhouse International

Introduction

Welcome to Reduce Mental Health Stigma in the Workplace. 5 ways to save money and support your local community. I look forward to sharing with you my vision of how organisations of any size can benefit from employing people who participate in The Clubhouse's Transitional Employment Program (TEP), and other programmes like it. I know so many people like myself who live with mental health issues and are highly motivated to contribute. I've written this book to help bring people like us together with the business community. It is my intention to serve as an ambassador for the integration of people with mental health issues alongside colleagues without mental health issues in the workplace.

I chose to write this book because I recognised that, as someone who went from having no mental health problems to living with permanent cognitive impairment, subsequent depression and suicidal thoughts as a result of brain tumour surgery, I am uniquely positioned to bridge the divide between those with and those without mental health issues. I know what it feels like to start out in life as a 'normal' person, then lose my friends, my job, and everything I knew due to mental health problems.

One of my biggest takeaways from my long journey to self-acceptance is that stigma against people with mental illness persists mostly due to silence surrounding the topic, and this serves no one. In a culture where the media – both news and 'entertainment' – depicts those with mental health issues as people to be feared, the only hope we have to end this stigma is to engage in honest 'cross-cultural' dialogue. That is, stigma will only end when people who do not suffer from mental illness have regular opportunities to interact, in a mutually-safe space, with those of us who do. The Clubhouse model of work-ordered day and workplace integration has been highly successful in providing such opportunities to the employees of those companies that have partnered with the programmes. Participants on both sides testify to the many ways in which this programme has enriched their lives.

I believe that if models like Clubhouse International's Transitional Employment Program are more widely adopted, the conversation around mental illness will evolve rapidly to the great benefit of not only those of us with mental health challenges, but our 'normal' colleagues as well. Until this happens, the media will retain the power to shape people's perceptions of us, and we will continue to experience challenges to economic self-sufficiency as well as social isolation and prejudice. Like most illnesses, mental health problems can be effectively treated in a variety of ways, but the stigma associated with them prevents many people from seeking the help they need, sending them on a downward spiral of despair. This is an unnecessary tragedy, and we must work to banish the stigma against mental health problems if we want to create a culture in which people feel comfortable asking for help.

By reading this book, you are choosing to be part of the solution, and I wish to thank you on behalf of everyone with mental health challenges, as well as their loved ones and other allies. Together, we can leave stigma towards mental health challenges behind, and step hand in hand into a future full of mutual respect and enrichment for all.

Sincerely,
Jeffy Wong

Chapter 1
It's Time to End the Stigma Against Mental Health Problems

"Imagine if you got blamed for having cancer."
– Message on a banner at a gathering in support of
ending the stigma against mental health problems

At the heart of stigma is a set of unquestioned beliefs and assumptions about what it means to have mental health problems. These beliefs suggest that mentally ill people have nothing valuable to offer, and contribute only chaos and difficulties to work and relationships. These beliefs have persisted from historic times, when mental illness was seen as a character flaw that earned sufferers the disdain of society at large. In those days, mental illness was viewed as a sin, not an illness that patients had no choice about, and as such they carried a heavy burden of shame. This shame led people to keep silent around the topic of mental health problems, explaining them away and denying any association whatever with the mentally ill. People with mental health problems were often sent by their families to residential institutions, where they lived out their days in isolation from the rest of society.

Although the institutional model has now fallen out of favour, the stigma persists, and it creates a perceived lack of support for both those living with mental health problems and their families. The subject of stigma itself is shrouded in obscurity, simply because people don't like to admit that they may harbour stigma themselves, however unconsciously. This is why I feel it's important to define the term 'stigma' in a way that makes clear what we are dealing with, so that we may 'know the enemy,' so to speak. I like the following definition from the British organisation Time to Change, whose mission is to end mental health discrimination:

Stigma is broadly defined as a collection of adverse and unfair beliefs. The stigma around mental health most often leads to the inaccurate and hurtful objectification of people as dangerous and incompetent. The shame and isolation associated with stigma prevents people from seeking the help necessary to live healthy and full lives.

Stigma is present in many forms that pervade every sphere of society. There is social stigma, which reflects how the general public view mental illness – this can be seen in the way the media portrays people with mental health problems. Then there is institutional stigma, in which people with mental health challenges face discrimination and injustice in their efforts to receive support and exercise their rights as citizens. Self-stigma can be devastating when individuals take on societal beliefs about their own lack of worth due to mental health problems. Finally, associative stigma can cause a person's friends and family to ostracize them in an effort to avoid the stigma of being associated with someone who suffers from mental illness. There are no doubt other forms that stigma takes, but these are some of its more common manifestations.

While there is a wide spectrum of experience with stigma among people with mental illness, my story can be considered fairly typical. I will now share it in an effort to illustrate the havoc that stigma can create both personally and socially.

The Enemy is Both Within and Without

I moved to England from Hong Kong at age 17, and was working as a credit controller when I began having unusual headaches. At first they were attributed to stress, but then I blacked out on the underground the day before my 31st birthday in 1998, and my life changed forever.

When an MRI was conducted at the hospital, doctors discovered a tumour situated on the frontal lobe of my brain, right between my eyebrows. The doctor told me, "Mr. Wong, you are not going home." When I blacked out again while in hospital, it was decided that an operation should be arranged urgently. The prospect of brain surgery was frightening, but at least the tumour was operable – I knew I had to go ahead with the surgery and hope for the best. I received the surgery two weeks following the discovery of the tumour.

I recovered well physically, but it soon became apparent that my cognitive function had been seriously impacted. The most obvious difference was in my speech patterns, since it now took much longer for me to find the right words to express what I wished to convey. Post-surgery, I also found it extremely challenging to carry out the ordinary tasks of daily life – my capacity for memory, planning and organizing, had suffered a major blow. Immediately after surgery, my body felt very heavy and I could hardly move. Doing anything required special effort, but certain mental functions that had been effortless before were especially taxing. When the nurses or doctors asked me questions like what is my name, do I know where I am, or what date is it today, sometimes I could hear the answer in my mind but couldn't say it, or worse, sometimes I just didn't understand what they were saying and felt confused. It was clear I would need a great deal of help adapting to my new life.

I was referred to a neuro-rehabilitation course run by Wolfson Centre, where they specialised in the treatment of head injury. I found this course very beneficial because I met other people in a similar situation, and we were able to swap stories. The course had many different aspects, such as helping participants understand what had happened, emotional aspects, and organising our thoughts. It taught me how to present myself and how to cope with the outside world to some degree. I learned that people are not interested in my medical history; they are only interested in whether I can do the task at hand. They just want to know things like whether I can turn up on time and remember what to do. This helped me to manage social situations more effectively, but since I now had difficulty with word-retrieval, I still struggled to communicate.

My parents had flown in from Hong Kong to spend two weeks with me following my surgery, but when they left I was still a long way from independence. Looking back now, I see that none of us had been sufficiently prepared for what my cognitive impairment would mean for my ability to re-integrate into the world. I didn't really know what to expect, and neither did anyone close to me; we just assumed that I would regain function over time, since no one had suggested otherwise. What's more, I was still deeply identified with being the person that I had been pre-surgery; no one had prepared me for just how difficult it would be psychologically to accept my altered capabilities. After surgery, I felt like a stranger in someone else's life, no longer able to fulfil the roles and responsibilities of the person I had been before the tumour. This set me up for a painful cycle of anger, denial, and depression that ultimately resulted in the loss of my job, my home, and perhaps most crucially, my social support network. My friends slowly drifted away; they just didn't have the patience to interact with this new person who took so long to speak and didn't have the same personality they remembered. For a long time, my only regular contact with others was a weekly phone call with my parents.

For many months after the surgery, I struggled with the basic tasks of daily life. For example, it took great effort for me to remember to put water in the kettle before I switched it on. I forced myself to go shopping despite my crippling depression, knowing that if I didn't I would die of starvation, and then what would be the point of surviving a brain tumour? It was as if I wandered alone in a desolate desert landscape, without a soul to share my struggles with. I just went on blindly looking for water, to build on the desert metaphor, until finally I started to ask, why should I continue to struggle like this? I began to experience suicidal thoughts as more and more time passed without any sign of improvement.

As time went on, the shame and anger I felt towards myself increased. I struggled to accept the fact that from now on, certain things that had been easy for me before would require extreme concentration. Looking back now, I see that I was in the throes of a major identity crisis, believing that I was alone in my struggle. I remember one occasion in particular when I needed to catch a train. I knew which platform to go to, and I knew what time to expect the train, but another train bound for a different destination ended up arriving at that time, and I boarded it. When I realized my mistake I was so angry and upset with myself, I could hardly function. My disability presented enough of a challenge, but I made it many times worse with the harsh judgement that I held towards myself for being apparently 'less-than' my former self. I had not yet learnt that who we are is so much more than what we are, or are not, able to do, and I struggled to believe that I still had worth as a human being, despite my disability.

Healing the Wounds of Stigma in Community

After I left hospital following the rehabilitation course, I returned to my old flat, but was forced to move a few months later when the landlord sold the property. Moving house was overwhelming for me, because a major aspect of my disability is difficulty with directions. The stress of not knowing my neighbours and needing to find my way around a new neighbourhood caused a severe outbreak of the eczema I had suffered from since childhood, landing me in hospital again. It was during this stay that I got what I consider to be a lucky break, in the form of a staff therapist who referred me to a support group for stroke survivors called Different Strokes, since recovery from stroke is similar to recovery from brain surgery. I joined the group and attended meetings every week for many years, becoming group coordinator after a few years and even holding a part-time paid position as regional coordinator for a time, until a lack of funding caused the position to be cut.

I had enjoyed this job, which involved visiting all of the London Different Strokes groups and helping with their development. I also attended several conferences representing Different Strokes. In the supportive environment created by this group, I began to once again feel I had a reason for living. I contributed to a newsletter called Disabilities Times, and even organised a conference for stroke survivors in 2006. It was incredibly rewarding to feel I was making a difference for others who were experiencing challenges similar to my own.

When the job with Different Strokes ended, I set out immediately to find another way to fill my time productively. That was when I began to spend more time at the day centre for mental health patients that I had been referred to in Brixton, South London, which was called the Effra Centre. Going to this centre each day gave me a much-needed reason to get out of bed in the morning as well as a square meal each day, and helped me overcome the depression that had taken hold. Using the skills I learnt at Disabilities Times, I eventually created a quarterly user-led newsletter for the centre entitled Inside Effra. The newsletter was a vehicle for members to contribute stories, poems, and other forms of self-expression. It was for the members, by the members, and we were especially pleased to know the newsletter was being distributed to various heads of departments in local council and hospital trusts. It helped us to feel valued, and this made all the difference.

The Clubhouse Transitional Employment Program

Eventually, the Effra Centre closed down and was replaced by the Mosaic Clubhouse, and I have been attending that centre from Monday to Friday every week since. A major difference between the new Clubhouse and the old Effra Centre was the work-ordered nature of the Clubhouse's programs. The Effra Centre had provided activities and social engagement, but the Clubhouse's emphasis on meaningful work added value for me and the other members. Not only did this program offer more purpose and structure, it had the potential to lead to real work opportunities, and this is what really sets it apart.

The award-winning Clubhouse model provides a place where people with serious mental illness can engage in a work-ordered life. It is founded on the understanding that the needs and capabilities of people in recovery from mental illness vary not only from individual to individual, but throughout each person's recovery timeline. Clubhouse staff are trained to support Clubhouse members in functioning at the maximum level of independence that that individual can sustain. In the Transitional Employment Program (TEP), members are accompanied at work by Clubhouse staff, who help them develop effective strategies for coping with the work environment so they can eventually fulfil a job's requirements independently. This relieves employers of the need to devote additional resources to accommodating the Clubhouse employee, while giving the employee personalised support that empowers them to test the limits of their independence in a safe environment.

Laying aside the assumption that all persons with mental health problems are the same is a prerequisite to creating an open dialogue in which stigma can be dismantled. By seeing each person with mental illness as the individual they are, we create a foundation on which everyone can build a successful and independent life.

Chapter 2
Stigma Holds Us All Back

"As long as stigma exists, it prevents society as a whole from incorporating these illnesses into a dialogue...
When we just open up the conversation and begin speaking about it, it's amazing what can happen."
– From an introductory video for the American advocacy organization Bring Change 2 Mind, co-founded by actor Glenn Close

I've written this book to encourage business owners to consider employing motivated people with mental health challenges via proven models such as Clubhouse International's Transitional Employment Program. My experience with the Clubhouse has shown me the difference that it makes for people with mental health problems to have access to meaningful work and a sense of contribution. I would even venture to say that the opportunity to work is one of the single most effective ways we have to combat the social isolation and depression that too many of us suffer with. It gives us a sense of contribution that is vital to our long-term wellbeing.

There's no question that going to work is good for people with mental health challenges, but the benefits are far from one-sided. Good executives know that keeping morale high is key to the bottom line, and no one is more grateful for work than people who have been denied economic opportunity in the past. This is why I believe that stigma against people with mental health challenges not only holds them back, but also puts unnecessary limits on what is possible for organisations. There is so much to be said for simply opening a dialogue on these topics, and that is exactly what this book aims to do.

Getting to Know an Invisible Disability

We are fortunate to live in a time when there is growing agreement that stigma is unfair and unjustified. The Information Age has allowed anti-stigma messages to reach a larger audience than ever before, and each year there seems to be more openness than there was previously. There are wonderful groups worldwide that are working to end stigma in a variety of areas including mental illness, and their messages seem to be getting through now more than ever. I've also observed that the reduction in stigma against particular sub-groups has coincided with an overall trend towards greater transparency and the reduction of prejudice in both the business and political spheres.

More value than ever is being placed on the creation of transparent and positive organisational cultures that welcome everyone, and this has been reinforced by comprehensive anti-discrimination hiring laws in many nations. Sweeping legislation has been put in place in many countries to protect the rights of people with a variety of medical disabilities. However, in too many places, support systems and reasonable accommodations for employees with mental illness have still not caught up with those available to people with physical disabilities, and I would like to see this change in my lifetime.

Those of us with mental health challenges face an added layer of discrimination due to the fact that our disabilities are not immediately visible. Many times people have told me that I make coping with the changes I've dealt with look easy, but this is far from the truth. I know I am lucky to be healthy physically, but sometimes I still catch myself thinking that life would be easier if people could tell that I was different just by looking at me. Because my disability is invisible, I frequently experience a change in people's perception of me in real time as we attempt to communicate. This is what dealt the worst blow to my self-esteem after my surgery: being first perceived as "normal", and then being on the receiving end of misunderstanding or stigma when my disability was discovered.

While I have learnt to function quite well in many ways, the challenges I face with communication continue to dog me. For example, if I get lost in the city and can't explain myself – both of which have become frequent occurrences as a result of my disability – the people I ask for help often assume I'm a drunk and ignore me. However, if I start by telling them about my cognitive and word-finding difficulties, they will perceive me immediately through the lens of stigma, which also makes them avoid me. Either way I lose; I am either perceived as drunk, or I am pushed away due to stigma. This is why it is so crucial for people with mental illness to have a place like the Clubhouse to go to, where we feel safe and accepted just as we are.

It's my dream to see the day when the general public has sufficient understanding of mental illness to know how to respond sensitively when they encounter people like me. The Clubhouse staff members know because of their training that we need compassion and support, not judgement. If everyone understood the truth about mental illness the way they do, stigma and the shame it brings would quickly disappear. I believe that workplace integration represents the best chance we have to make this dream a reality.

Challenging Myths About Mental Illness

It's wonderful to attend conferences featuring speakers like Raymond Aaron, and see so many people beginning to re-frame fear as False Evidence Appearing Real. The appearance of memes like this in the culture signals a new awareness that we can question old fear-based beliefs, and replace them with ones based on love and inclusion. This is a very heartening and long-overdue development.

A good place to start dismantling stigma is to dissect and disprove some of the most prevalent myths surrounding mental illness. One such myth is that mental health problems are rare, when in fact 1 in 4 people in the United Kingdom will experience some kind of mental health problem in a given year. We all know at least one person who contends with mental ill health in one way or another, and it is only the silence that stigma creates that causes us to believe otherwise. This silence is so destructive, because it prevents people from seeking help when they need it in an effort to avoid stigma from friends and family. Yet it serves no one when people feel they must face mental health challenges alone.

Myth #1: Mental Health Problems Are Rare

Fact: best estimates are that at least 1 in 4 people in the UK will suffer from mental health problems to some degree in any given year. To give you a more detailed picture of the prevalence of mental ill health in the UK population, I'd like to share some statistics from a survey that is done every seven years in England. The results of this survey are published by the Health and Social Care Information Centre under the title Adult Psychiatric Morbidity in England. Below are the numbers revealed by the most recent survey in 2009. Note that this survey is conducted only on people living at home, so these numbers do not include people with mental health problems who reside in hospitals or prisons:

Depression	2.6 in 100 people
Anxiety	4.7 in 100 people
Mixed anxiety and depression	9.7 in 100 people
Phobias	2.6 in 100 people
OCD	1.3 in 100 people
Panic disorder	1.2 in 100 people

Post traumatic stress disorder   3.0 in 100 people
Eating disorders   1.6 in 100 people

Some problems are asked about over a person's lifetime, rather than each year:

Suicidal thoughts   17 in 100 people
Self-harm   3 in 100 people

Estimates for bipolar disorder, schizophrenia and personality disorders are also usually described over a person's lifetime, rather than each year. Estimates for the number of people with these diagnoses vary, but the most commonly reported figures are:

Personality disorders   3 to 5 people in every 100
Bipolar disorder   1 to 3 people in every 100
Schizophrenia   1 to 3 people in every 100

From these statistics we can estimate that perhaps 10% of the UK population will directly experience challenges to their mental health at some point in their lives. This means we will all have friends, family or colleagues who suffer from some form of mental ill health, now or in the past or future. Mental health is an invisible epidemic, and ignoring this epidemic will not make it go away. Like most diseases, mental health problems can be treated and managed once they are diagnosed. Another similarity with other health problems is that the prognosis and treatment options are better the earlier mental health problems are diagnosed. A major consequence of stigma is that it causes people who suffer a mental health setback to delay seeking treatment, negatively impacting every aspect of their lives.

Myth #2: People With Mental Illness Can't or Won't Work

Another destructive myth is that people with mental health problems are not willing or able to work, but the fact is that we probably all work with someone who has experienced some degree of mental health challenges at some point in their life. No one expects someone who has had a severe accident or emergency surgery to go back to work right away because we know they need time to recover, but at least in these cases it is usually assumed that recovery is possible. Recovery from mental ill health may not be complete but with treatment can be controlled.

Clubhouse International's worldwide network of Transitional Employment Programmes provides proof that people in recovery from mental ill health can be a major asset to employers large and small. Clubhouse members must reach certain milestones in their recovery in order to qualify for these programmes, just as an injured pro athlete must regain a certain level of fitness before he can be allowed to play again. While that athlete is in recovery, attending the gym and doing physiotherapy, all he thinks about is getting back in the game. In the same way, most people who have suffered setbacks in life due to mental health problems are highly motivated to work – they just need training, encouragement, and the right support to get back in the game of economic self-sufficiency.

Myth #3: People with mental health problems are violent and unpredictable

This unfortunate myth persists despite the fact that people with mental ill health are actually far more likely to be victims of violence than perpetrators of it. It is a gross misperception fed by a news and entertainment media that is obsessed with telling violent and extreme stories, rather than those that reflect the truth. In over twelve years placing hundreds of workers through its TEPs, Mosaic Clubhouse has never once had to deal with inappropriate behaviour by its members in their workplaces. Just as good doctors don't let people who've had surgery return to work too early, Clubhouse TEPs are reserved only for those members who have demonstrated their readiness to work via their daily participation in Clubhouse life. Mosaic's TEP track record speaks much louder than the media's voice of negativity.

The End of Stigma Starts At Work

We know that direct social contact between people with mental health problems and those with "normal" mental function is the best way to challenge stigma and change public attitudes, and the workplace presents a natural opportunity to foster this connection. Stigma in any context is fed by ignorance and silence, which reinforce each other. Therefore, the way to dispel it is for people with and without mental illness to stop avoiding each other and break the silence. People need to talk about what mental illness is and is not, and they need to do it in a safe space where both parties can air their feelings and concerns without fear of judgement. Stigma begins to melt away almost immediately in such an environment.

As we've discussed, paid work is one of the most effective ways for people with mental illness to create a sense of meaning and fulfilment in their lives. Yet the beliefs and misconceptions that are inherent in stigma prevent many employers from hiring those with mental health problems. In recognition of the need for change, the Clubhouse organisation created a revolutionary program that addresses the most common concerns employers have, while also providing additional advantages. The Mosaic Clubhouse alone has helped several hundred people in the London area return to work, and the numbers are growing. These accomplishments are not insignificant if, like many people in business, you are fiscally conservative and interested in reducing the cost of government programmes that support people with disabilities. Consider the following:

- People with severe, long-term mental health problems who are given intensive support to return to the workplace report fewer and shorter subsequent hospital stays than people receiving standard mental health services.
- The financial costs of the adverse effects of mental illness on people's quality of life are significant every year in England. Wider costs to the national economy in terms of welfare benefits, lost productivity at work, etc. are even more substantial.
- The costs of mental health services can be reduced by half when people with severe mental health problems are supported into mainstream employment.
- In New York City, where the original Clubhouse known as Fountain House is located, a two-week

hospital stay costs $28,000. For this amount, Fountain House can secure a member's housing for an entire year, plus access to community services, health care, education, employment and social support.

In addition to the fiscal savings that workplace-integration programmes for people with mental illness offer to businesses, such programmes also help build valuable social capital as part of a positive corporate culture. Ines Gnaulati of CNBC Europe, a long-time partner with Mosaic Clubhouse, had this to say about the company's experience with Clubhouse TEP participants:

I have had the pleasure of working with a number of people from Mosaic over the years. Each person brings something new to the position of Library Assistant. Their flexibility and enthusiastic approach to their work is evident in the quality and quantity of the tasks they carry out. The role they provide is important to the daily running of our media library.

Ms. Gnaulati and others like her have directly experienced working alongside participants in Mosaic's TEP programme, and this has given them a permanent ability to separate the myths of mental illness from the reality. As with any stigma against a group that is perceived as 'other,' the stigma against those in recovery from mental ill health is best dispelled through direct social contact, and the workplace can provide a ready-made safe container within which such contact can occur. That's why I believe that the end of stigma against those with mental health challenges begins at work, and as an executive or business owner, I hope you will consider becoming part of the solution by partnering with your local Clubhouse's TEP programme.

A Closer Look at the Clubhouse Model

Internationally, the Clubhouse organisation has set the standard for supported workplace integration of people with serious mental health challenges. The accomplishments of Clubhouse International were recognised in 2014 with the Conrad N. Hilton Humanitarian Prize, which at 1.5 million dollars is the world's largest humanitarian prize. The foundation presents this award each year to a different organisation, in recognition of extraordinary work to relieve human suffering. Steven M. Hilton, president and CEO of the foundation, issued the following statement to accompany the 2014 award:

The Fountain House / Clubhouse International program of social relationships and meaningful work has literally saved thousands of lives over the past 66 years. Its program is a beacon of hope for those living with mental illness who are too often consigned to lives of homelessness, imprisonment, social stigma and isolation... Its work demonstrates that we can unshackle those with mental disorders and stigma and embrace them as productive independent people with talents and contributions important to society.

By now, you know that the Clubhouse's Transitional Employment Programs (TEPs) provide major benefits to people living with mental health problems. Enlightened business leaders call this 'building social capital.' However, the fact that a company like Dow Jones has employed over 360 Clubhouse members in New York, London, and Tokyo to date suggests that the impact on financial capital must be at least as profound as the social impact. So how exactly does the TEP ensure that this value is provided? The answer is encapsulated in Mosaic Clubhouse's mission statement, which reads as follows:

Mosaic Clubhouse is an independent charity that develops partnerships with employers to increase their social capital and save them money. We do this by assuming the management, including recruitment, training, regular supervision and support of entry-level jobs. We use employment as our tool in assisting the recovery of people from mental ill health. After six to nine months, we support one employee to progress, ideally into their own job, then we offer the same opportunity to another person. We cover any absences and manage the transition from one employee to another smoothly and efficiently. We are part of an international network of Clubhouses that are accredited against 36 recovery-focused standards.

Simply put, the program essentially offloads entry level hiring, supervision, training, and even health coverage responsibilities for entry-level positions from a company's human resources department. This frees up the significant resources that were formerly locked up in dealing with turnover, in addition to guaranteeing perfect attendance on the job. The Clubhouse staff screen, train, and provide on-going support to potential job candidates, allowing them to eventually become able to perform their duties independently. Businesses of all sizes are drawn to the programme in recognition of the resources that it can save them, all while doing good for the community. The Clubhouse TEP programme provides businesses with an opportunity to 'do good and do well' to a remarkable degree, in over 30 countries around the world. The more the business community takes advantage of these programmes, the more money will be saved, and the faster the stigma against the mentally ill will dissolve amidst positive daily interactions with healthy colleagues over time.

Chapter 3
A Return to Wholeness

"When I received my diagnosis, I dedicated myself to education and advocacy - the tools of survival. Surrender was my greatest asset. Not defeat, but willingness. It was time to seek out solutions to problems that I didn't know I had."
– Henry Boy Jenkins

We all know that human beings are social animals. Indeed, meaningful contact with others of our kind is so crucial to our well-being that babies who don't receive enough loving attention fail to thrive, and social isolation is considered a serious risk factor for morbidity and mortality among the elderly. Likewise, the social isolation that too often accompanies mental ill health is one of the most destructive consequences that people experience from their mental health problems. I know that personally, I became much more susceptible to depression, paranoia, and even severe eczema outbreaks when I experienced social isolation prior to becoming a Clubhouse member. Many other members that I've spoken with share my view that the safe environment for social interaction provided at

Clubhouses is the foundation that makes the rest of the organisation's programmes so effective.

This core principle goes back to the formation of Fountain House, the original Clubhouse in New York City, over 60 years ago. Here is a brief description of how the Clubhouse model came about, taken from The Conrad N. Hilton Foundation's press release accompanying their $1.5 million award to Clubhouse International in 2014. You will see that positive social interaction was the glue that brought the first members together:

Fountain House/Clubhouse International started in the early 1940s at Rockland State Hospital in Orangeburg, New York. Seven patients formed a self-help group that met in a hospital '"club room" to prepare themselves to be discharged and cope with the challenges of finding shelter and work and dealing with relationships and inevitable relapses. Soon after leaving the hospital, they began to meet on the steps of the New York City Public Library to re-create the Clubhouse experience, believing that it would sustain their recovery, provide a mutual support system and ultimately lead to changing society's perception of people living with mental illness. They called it the "We Are Not Alone Society" which became Fountain House in

1948, named for its West 47th Street building that had a fountain in its garden.

It was her experience volunteering at Fountain House that inspired actor Glenn Close to start the US-based campaign known as BringChange2Mind, whose mission is to end the stigma and discrimination surrounding mental illness. She also nominated Clubhouse International for the Conrad N. Hilton Prize prior to 2014. In the same press release mentioned above, Ms. Close shares her enthusiasm for the Clubhouse model as follows:

I have been moved by the fact that Fountain House purposefully depends on people with mental illness for its daily operation and future, from answering phones to designing and running programs, to serving on the board of directors. Shared responsibility builds self-esteem and alleviates the stigma and isolation that so often haunt people with mental disorders.

Like Ms. Close, those seven founding fathers and mothers of Fountain House understood that despite the severe stigma that society greeted them with, they were not 'bad' or 'evil' people, but recovering from illness just like someone with tuberculosis or diabetes. They had been ill, and they knew that their illness would likely affect them to one degree or another for the remainder of their lives, but they refused to see themselves as lesser human beings because of it. With the support of each other and the hospital staff, they had begun the recovery process, and learned how to manage their symptoms just like anyone with a chronic illness. Yet because their illnesses afflicted them primarily at the mental level, they knew they could not expect the same treatment by society that asthmatics or recovering cancer patients received. Instead, they were met with suspicion and ill will by most people, and were sometimes even rejected by their own family and friends.

Because of this, they knew they would have to rely on each other for mutual support, and they did so with great success. When they realized how much this support group had helped each of them in their recovery, they opened the doors of Fountain House to all persons in recovery from mental illness who wished to heal, and a worldwide movement was born. Fountain House was unique at the time as a programme for recovery founded by and for those with mental health problems. As such, it was guided by a mission of empowerment from the beginning, in contrast to the condescension that often pervaded the mental institutions of the time.

Support That Recognizes Wholeness

One of the most painful aspects of living with mental health problems is constantly being perceived by others as somehow defective or 'less than' a healthy person. This is an aspect of stigma that affects us internally as well, as I related in an earlier chapter when I spoke of the identity crisis I experienced following my surgery. There is nothing worse than feeling that you are a failure as a human being, and that you have been permanently robbed of the ability to ever make a valuable contribution to society again. It's enough to drive many people to despair, and the way that the Clubhouse model addresses this specific issue is largely responsible for the positive recognition it has received in the international mental health care community.

The Clubhouse model rejects the pervasive view that people with mental health problems have nothing to contribute. Instead, it views them as whole, valuable individuals who are capable of much more than they may have thought possible. Staff recognise that many people with mental health problems become accustomed to viewing themselves as failures, and that they therefore must be set up for success from the beginning in order to rebuild their self-esteem. Clubhouse members are expected to contribute to the work required to run the

Clubhouse alongside staff members, but they are only assigned tasks that they feel confident undertaking, and which staff members feel certain they can succeed at. There is a clear recognition that every accomplishment made by a Clubhouse member is hard-won, and therefore worthy of celebration, and that every contribution members make is valuable and important to the Clubhouse's operation.

In the Clubhouse environment, there is simply no such thing as failure, and that is why becoming a Clubhouse member is so transformative for people affected by mental health problems. In the supportive, accepting environment that Clubhouses provide, people with mental health problems are given manageable ways to make a contribution, and as a result they begin to feel whole again. It is wonderful to watch, and as the recent award from the Hilton Foundation attests, it is one of the most effective ways to facilitate real recovery from mental health problems.

Whole People Want to Work

By now, I hope you are beginning to see that the way Clubhouse day centres operate directly prepares members to enter the workforce. Only people who wish to make as full a recovery as possible of their mental health become Clubhouse members, and only those members whom staff believe to be sufficiently recovered are offered the opportunity to participate in the centre's Transitional Employment Program (TEP). Because of this, every Clubhouse member who participates in the TEP is highly motivated to succeed in the positions you hire them for.

The centre I attend in London is Mosaic Clubhouse; their TEP operates on a principle of seamless integration between the work-ordered structure of the centre and outside employment. The work that Clubhouse members engage in at their respective centres is similar to work they might perform on an actual job site. Within the Clubhouse members are fully supported in an environment that helps them regain old skills and acquire new ones in a manageable way. Once members achieve a certain level of independence within the Clubhouse setting, they are then given the option of taking temporary positions through the TEP with that Clubhouse's partner organisations.

Positions are typically designed to occupy members for 15 – 20 hours per week over 6 – 9 months, with the Clubhouse providing a steady stream of entry-level employees fully trained and supported by Clubhouse staff at no cost to the company. Ideally, Clubhouse members eventually become capable of performing a job independently, at which point partner organisations may choose to hire them permanently. Clubhouse staff members go to great lengths to ensure that members are matched with positions that they are poised to succeed in, knowing that this benefits the member, the company, and the reputation of the Clubhouse approach. They even provide no-cost consulting services to help organisations design their entry-level positions to match the needs and capabilities of the member in question. They perform adaptive assessments on behalf of Clubhouse members in much the same way that consultants who work to make workplaces accessible for physically disabled employees perform their assessments, and they do this despite the fact that employers are not yet legally required to make such adjustments.

Essentially, the Clubhouse International charitable organisation funds efforts by Clubhouse branches around the world to make workplaces accessible for people with mental health challenges, in a way that resembles what companies are legally required to do under the physical disability laws that have been passed in many countries. Through the efforts of Clubhouses around the world, hundreds of people with mental health challenges have been successfully re-integrated into the workforce in a way that benefits both members and the companies they work for. We can only hope that in time, governments will recognise that people with mental health challenges also deserve to have laws put in place to protect their equal rights in the workplace and beyond. Until then, the Clubhouse model will continue to set the standard for how workplace equality can be achieved for persons with mental health challenges in communities worldwide.

Recovering Our Wholeness Together

It's simple really: when people are supported in returning to wholeness and regaining self-esteem, they want to work. Now that they have recovered, they want to live their recovery by making a meaningful contribution to the world, in whatever way they can. The process of recovery is hard work, so why would someone undertake it if they weren't determined to increase their sense of meaningful contribution and independence? As the woman from the CNBC London Office said in the previous chapter, Clubhouse members whom you employ through the TEP will be some of the most motivated and positive people that you will ever hire at the entry level. They will never take their job for granted, nor forget what a privilege it is to be able to make a contribution to society. People in recovery from mental health problems are whole, and they want to work. It may even be that their positive attitude inspires an increase in morale among your other employees, and that's always good for business!

My colleagues often tell me that they would never have realised I had a brain injury if I didn't tell them – that they would attribute my difficulty finding words to English being my second language, for example. They don't know how hard I've worked to learn to cope with my disability, and how much it means to me to hear them say that. Some of them have even told me that they find my story of recovery inspiring, and that I should share my message somehow, so here we are! This just goes to show you that daily interaction in the workplace between those unaffected by mental health problems and those living with them is a great way to dispel stigma. Not only do we gain a sense of acceptance and belonging, but our colleagues gain inspiration through our stories of overcoming adversity with patience, determination, and the ability to accept help. It's a real win-win.

I know that the valuable support I received in my recovery at Mosaic Clubhouse is the reason people now view me this way, and it's my passion to help others affected by mental health problems achieve this sense of fulfilment and belonging. I hope you will join me in support of

Clubhouse International, because I am living proof that this model works.

Chapter 4
Empowerment Through Inter-dependence

"Man often becomes what he believes himself to be. If I keep on saying to myself that I cannot do a certain thing, it is possible that I may end by really becoming incapable of doing it. On the contrary, if I have the belief that I can do it, I shall surely acquire the capacity to do it even if I may not have it at the beginning."
— Mahatma Gandhi

The award-winning Clubhouse model of recovery from mental ill health is founded on the belief that we are all interdependent, whether we realise it or not. In recognition of this, each Clubhouse provides members and staff alike with an opportunity to create fulfilling and productive lives by giving deliberate expression to this inter-dependence. While staff do receive comprehensive training for their roles, they are not clinicians and no therapy takes place on Clubhouse grounds. What does happen is that people who wish to take responsibility for their recovery from mental ill health make an active

41

contribution to the running of the Clubhouse community, and staff support them in doing so.

Clubhouses are best defined as community centres, and as such, they are run principally by and for their members. They are deliberately understaffed in order to allow members to take maximum responsibility for most of the day-to-day tasks involved in running their centre. In any Clubhouse around the world, you will find members and staff working side-by-side to create and run a community whose goal is the support and enrichment of people in recovery from mental ill health. This model is founded on the principle of equality, and a natural expression of this is inter-dependence. Staff are present to provide support as needed, but it is the opportunity to support each other in the roles and responsibilities of membership that does the most for members' self-esteem. The success of the Clubhouse model in helping people gain greater financial and functional independence is a testament to the fact that recognizing and fostering interdependence supports those in recovery in achieving greater independence as well.

When a new member first walks into a Clubhouse, perhaps feeling a bit nervous or uncertain, it is often the other members who go to the greatest lengths to make them feel comfortable and welcome. Knowing that their fellow members are also in recovery makes new members feel more confident learning new things and trying new roles, sometimes for the first time in years. Many new members have not felt valued for who they are in a long time, and for them, joining a Clubhouse represents a major breakthrough in rebuilding their self-esteem. That's certainly been my experience, and I know it will resonate for others as well.

The Clubhouse model uses a focus on interdependence to remind members that we all have valuable skills and talents to contribute. By believing in our worth and focusing on what we can do instead of what we can't, we help each other gain a foothold on a life of fulfilment and productivity that too many of us believed we'd never have. This benefits not only members, but society at large, as people who would have been given up on in times past begin to make a contribution once again.

Features of A Clubhouse Community

By now, you've heard a bit about the Transitional Employment Program offered at most Clubhouses, but what are the features of daily life at a Clubhouse? How do the spheres of daily activity that make up a Clubhouse community intersect and synergise to create a space in which people can build the strength, motivation, and skills to reclaim their lives from the ravages of mental ill health? Of course, as with any community, the individual threads that compose the larger tapestry of a Clubhouse are too varied and numerous to list individually, but a closer look at some of the core features of the Clubhouse model can give us a sense of what makes it unique. Here is a list of the defining characteristics of a Clubhouse, taken from the Clubhouse International website:

- A work-ordered day in which the talents and abilities of members are recognized and utilized within the Clubhouse;

- Participation in consensus-based decision making regarding all important matters relating to the running of the Clubhouse;

- Opportunities to obtain paid employment in the local labour market through a Clubhouse-created Transitional Employment Program. In addition, members participate in Clubhouse-supported and independent programs;

- Assistance in accessing community-based educational resources;

- Access to crisis intervention services when needed;

- Evening/weekend social and recreational events; and

- Assistance in securing and sustaining safe, decent and affordable housing.

As we've already discussed, Clubhouses operate on a principle of equality, and this is reflected in the consensus-based decision making model that they adhere to. Also, there is no part of any Clubhouse building that is off-limits to members, in recognition that they share the same responsibility as staff for every aspect of clubhouse affairs. When they join, members are given a choice of where they wish to concentrate their efforts in support of the community, whether it be via preparing, serving, and selling food, maintaining the building and grounds, or helping with more administrative tasks. These various avenues of participation correspond to real-world career tracks, thus laying the groundwork for employment for any member who wishes to pursue it – and the majority do.

New members are trained to carry out tasks for the Clubhouse community from their very first day, and for many this will be the first time they have worked in years.

Members choose an area of work that appeals to them, and staff trains them to perform it independently. While the primary aim of this approach is to improve member self-esteem and fulfilment rather than to make them employable, it does also have the added benefit of preparing people to participate in the TEP should they choose to do so. It is understood that some days will be better than others on the journey of recovery, but the intention and commitment to work and serve the community is what qualifies someone to become a Clubhouse member.

As noted above, daily life in Clubhouses is work-ordered, meaning that the majority of activities take place between 9 AM and 5 PM daily Monday - Friday, with occasional social or educational opportunities being offered outside those times. In particular, Clubhouses often provide activities for members during holiday times, when those in recovery from mental ill health tend to experience the most isolation and lack of support. Planning these activities is an aspect of Clubhouse work that many members greatly enjoy, because people who have struggled with mental ill health know first-hand how important social engagement is to the recovery process. There are game nights, barbecues, presentations from local artists and organisations, and the list goes on.

While it's true that a Clubhouse can connect members to services such as crisis intervention and affordable housing when needed, these things are secondary to the main purpose of a Clubhouse, which is to facilitate recovery from mental ill health by giving members a place to learn, grow, contribute, and support each other. For many, just knowing that there is a place they'll always be able to go to for support, acceptance, and connection is life-changing. As one member put it in her testimonial, the knowledge that the Clubhouse community will always be there for her is what gives her the courage to overcome the obstacles she faces in life, because now, for the first time, she knows she is not alone. I can personally resonate with this sentiment, and I know that many other Clubhouse members can as well. Words can't describe how important it is for those of us living with mental ill health to know that we are not alone.

The following excerpt from the Clubhouse International website provides a clear description of what makes the Clubhouse model stand out from other approaches to mental health rehabilitation:

Although Fountain House started more than fifty years ago and has been replicated more than four hundred times around the world, the Clubhouse concept is still a radically different way of working in the field of community mental health. Most programme models still focus on assessing a person's level of disability and limiting expectations based on that assessment. Most use teaching or treatment as the vehicle for providing rehabilitation. In a Clubhouse the expectations are high and mutual work, mutual relationships, and meaningful opportunities in the community are the vehicles of choice.

What is so unique and valuable about Clubhouses is that from the very first day, they focus on what's right with a person, not what's wrong with them. This may seem like a subtle distinction, but it makes all the difference not only for members, but for everyone who interacts with a Clubhouse community. Walking into a place like Mosaic Clubhouse does not feel like walking into a hospital, treatment centre, or government aid agency; it feels like walking into a vibrant community hub where quite simply, good things are happening, and the results that members achieve bear out this impression strongly.

Mosaic Clubhouse, a Model Community

At this stage, I feel it's time to give some attention to my own Clubhouse community, the Mosaic Clubhouse in London, UK. In the last week of 2014, we added to our list of honours a Collaboration Award given by the Lambeth Collaborative in partnership with the organisation Care Management Matters, which created it along with several other Third Sector Care awards. Here is what the judges for the Third Sector Care awards had to say about why they chose Mosaic Clubhouse for this accolade:

This organisation has a seamless approach where all individuals (staff and people with lived experience) are valued adults and where there is true equality in support. An organisation that does not see barriers but opportunities. An organisation that is solution-based. They link in early to support individuals with their own pathway. This organisation has developed a Clubhouse model which is dynamic, user-led and has excellent collaborations.

Elsewhere, they noted that Mosaic Clubhouse's "values and approach really illustrated where the strengths model of mental health and wellbeing (aspirations and confidence) can create meaningful futures." The timing of this award coincided auspiciously with the 20th anniversary of the Mosaic Clubhouse's opening on Effra Road in Brixton, a day that heralded a new era for me and the hundreds of other members who have become involved since. The quality of our community has attracted an array of high-quality partners to join forces with us, whether as TEP partners providing employment opportunities for members or in an educational or other supportive capacity.

For example, top-tier recruiting firm Harris Global has made its CV-preparation and job counselling services available to our members on a charitable basis. Alan Feast, the founder of the firm, has committed to this partnership because he has seen the effectiveness of the collaboration between Mosaic Clubhouse members and staff, as well as numerous local organisations and even local government. This has made it possible for a very high percentage of TEP participants at Mosaic to obtain and keep independent employment once they finish their placements, and this is something everyone can celebrate.

As a result of these achievements and more, we have become one of only 10 sites in the world where staff are trained, having passed our site inspections every three years with flying colours. This is a source of pride that every Clubhouse member and staff member is fully invested in. In its twenty-year history, Mosaic Clubhouse has repeatedly surpassed expectations of what a recovery community is capable of, becoming indispensable not only to those with mental ill health, but to the community at large. I am proud to be part of it, and I hope that more people in the business community will see in Mosaic a model of how recovery and business can enhance and support each other even more. The sky is the limit!

Chapter 5
Transitional Employment Programs: Good for Recovery and the Bottom Line

Our partnership with Fountain House has benefited our company as much as it has the members of Fountain House. We get highly motivated workers and the reward of making an impact on someone else's life.
- Leslie Harwood, Managing Director,
Newmark Grubb Knight Frank

By now, you have a good understanding of why the Clubhouse model works for people living with mental illness, and why the Transitional Employment Programs that are offered through Clubhouses are central to the model's effectiveness. In this chapter, we'll take a more in-depth look at the data that back up the successful experiences of hundreds of Clubhouse members the world over. What I find in my efforts to spread the word about the Clubhouse model is that, while the heart tends to understand the benefits of the Clubhouse approach quite readily, the head sometimes requires more convincing. This is only human nature, and I have written this book in an effort to convince more heads that in the idea that recovery from mental ill health and good business sense can enhance each other hand-in-hand.

Social and psychological researchers have long seen the value in community-based models for recovery from mental health problems, and have devoted considerable resources to researching what makes them so effective. These results have been presented at global health summits, and have been used to shape national mental-health policies in a number of countries, including the United Kingdom. While there are many approaches to community-based mental health care, the Clubhouse model has been shown to produce superior results in many cases. We will take a deeper look at the reasons for this in the pages to come.

Good For Recovery

It is a persistent and damaging myth that persons in recovery from mental ill health do not wish to work, even if they are capable of doing so. While it is true that many new Clubhouse members have been out of work for a time when they first join, sometimes for years, this is less due to a lack of will than it is to stigma, and a lack of adequate support for recovery. We know this because two studies published in 1999 and 2001 found that 70 – 90 % of people who were out of work as a result of severe mental health problems wanted to be employed (Grove, 1999; Secker & Seebohm, 2001). In study after study, the data shows conclusively that being in paid work is one of the most powerful factors influencing recovery from mental ill health. For example, a study published in 2006 ("Is Work Good for Your Health & Well-being?" by Gordon Waddell and A Kim Burton) concluded that supporting people with severe or enduring mental health problems to gain or stay in employment improves their prognosis significantly by breaking 'a downward spiral of unemployment, deterioration in mental health and consequent reduced chances of gaining employment.'

In light of this, it's clear that interventions are needed which can break this cycle by helping those in recovery from mental ill health to re-enter the work force for the long-term. In 2010 a charitable organisation called the King's Fund, which conducts research on the subject of how England's health care system can be improved, published a comprehensive report entitled Mental Health and the Productivity Challenge: Improving Quality and Value for Money in response to a looming budget crisis in the National Health Service (NHS). In a section entitled Providing Effective Employment Support, this report advocates for TEP – style employment programs as superior to other models. There is an excerpt below:

There is … clear evidence that certain approaches to supporting employment are more cost-effective than others. The individual placement and support (IPS) approach [eg., Clubhouse's TEP] has consistently been found to outperform traditional train-then-place or sheltered work schemes, and succeeds in helping more than half of its participants to return to employment .

The defining features of IPS are that people are supported to find competitive employment (as opposed to vocational training placements) as quickly as possible, and then provided with support and training when in post. The key principles are:

- Competitive employment is the primary goal
- Everyone who wants employment support is eligible for it
- Job search is rapid and consistent with individual preferences
- Employment specialists and clinical teams are co-located and work together [note that this is not a feature of the Clubhouse model, although Clubhouses do refer members to treatment when necessary]

- Tailored in-work support is available for as long as necessary
- Counselling on welfare benefits supports the individual through the transition from benefits to work

According to Sainsbury Centre for Mental Health Briefing 41 : The Economic and Financial Case for Supported Employment, the annual cost of implementing IPS across the NHS is estimated to be about 67 million. The current annual spend on day and employment services for people with mental health problems is 184 million. This suggests that a national roll-out of IPS could be afforded within existing budgets by diverting some resources from less effective models.

Evidence from "Relatively Inexpensive and Highly Cost-Effective Relative to Other Forms of Vocational Services" (Drake and Bond, 2008) suggests that one-third of IPS participants become regular workers, some of whom will no longer need state benefits. A further one-third become occasional workers. Both of these groups will enjoy higher incomes and greater independence and are likely to require fewer hospital admissions over time, thus reducing costs to the NHS in the long term. There is growing evidence that savings to the NHS alone could more than cover the cost of providing IPS.

As I mentioned in an earlier chapter, anyone who is in favour of reducing the cost of government can easily find reason to support TEP-style employment programmes for people with mental health problems. These studies and many others show that the numbers really do add up for both public- and private-sector service providers (and for partnerships between the two), as well as for those in recovery who are able to get back on their feet with supported work placements.

Good for the Bottom Line

We've now seen evidence for the efficiency of a TEP-style employment support model from a public health policy perspective, but what are the most compelling benefits of this type of programme for partner businesses? At the macro level, there are five principle benefits of TEPs for employers:

1. Pre-trained staff. The emphasis on a work-ordered day as a prerequisite for members' participation in a Clubhouse community ensures that people begin to build the skills they need to be employable from their first day at the centre. Whether they work in administration, education / outreach, or hospitality and horticulture, members are learning new skills and

honing old ones each day that they attend their Clubhouse. One of the guidelines that all Clubhouses must adhere to is that staff ratios must strike a balance between providing sufficient support for members, and ensuring that members' work is truly indispensable to the functioning of the Clubhouse. This creates an atmosphere of empowerment for members that quickly and effectively prepares them for outside work, even if they have previously been out of work for years. Members are only placed in TEPs once they've demonstrated the ability to cope with the work-ordered structure of daily Clubhouse life. They are recognised as being job-ready when their skills, interests, values and needs match the demands of a specific placement, and the values and needs of that placement's employer.

2. Guaranteed back-up staff in case of absence. An integral feature of the Clubhouse's supported employment programme is that Clubhouse staff commit to filling in for members who are unable to fulfil their placement as scheduled on any given day. This ensures that members have the flexibility to deal with the setbacks that can happen on the road to recovery from mental ill health without fear of losing their jobs. It recognises that the path of recovery is seldom linear, and that independence is rebuilt in

stages over time. This feature ensures that members can continue to cultivate job skills even as they take the time they need to heal.

3. A ready pool of candidates for part-time, entry-level positions. Human resource managers at firms large and small know what a headache it can be to keep part-time entry-level positions filled with qualified and motivated candidates. Many such managers testify to the relief they've found by partnering with their local Clubhouse to provide placements for TEPs. Now they can devote much more of their precious time and energy to other important matters, because they know that these crucial positions will be reliably filled.

4. No recruitment costs. With TEP, it is not necessary to advertise posts or interview as this is all taken care of by Clubhouse staff.

5. No sick or holiday pay. Because TEP placements are usually for no more than 15 to 20 hours of work per week, employers do not take on the responsibility of sick and holiday pay for people employed via these programmes. Additionally, even in countries whose health care systems are primarily ruled by the private

sector, many Clubhouse members receive public health care benefits due to their mental health problems.

Here is a more micro-level look at the many benefits enjoyed by companies that partner with Clubhouses to create TEPs:

1. The staff for TEP jobs are sourced and selected by the Clubhouse in question, which means that you will never need to find reliable workers and worry about staff turnover.

2. TEP jobs can be a cost-effective way to minimize the strain of covering entry-level tasks on other staff at the organisation.

3. TEP is fully supported; therefore the employer can be sure that there will be no drop in productivity during the changeover of staff or through the course of employment. Usually members transition to either another TEP position or independent employment after a period of 6 to 9 months; they are always replaced immediately since there is a waiting list in most locations for TEP placement.

4. Guaranteed 100% free absence coverage during any placement by Clubhouse staff.

5. Staff from Mosaic Clubhouse will provide a high level of supervision of the TEP employee, and support to both the employer and employee.

6. Each placement is maintained only if the member meets the work requirement of the employer.

7. New TEP placements are first performed by a staff worker so that an accurate assessment can be made of the job's requirements.

8. The Clubhouse can assist you to design and develop the TEP job so that it suits the needs of your organisation.

9. Mosaic staff that know and have worked the placement have primary responsibility for training the employee.

10. TEP placements increase an organisation's social capital and help them reduce the costs associated with entry-level employment.

If this is starting to sound too good to be true, be assured that Clubhouses around the world take pride in consistently exceeding the expectations of the companies they partner with for their Transitional Employment Programs (TEPs). The reasons they're able to do this are many, but the prominent business newspaper The Wall Street Journal summed it up beautifully in an article devoted to the benefits of TEPs for businesses, in which they concluded that TEPs are an example of how 'a good deed can be a good deal.' As I've said before, we know that TEPs have tremendous power to help people in recovery from mental ill health to rebuild their confidence, competence, and independence, but that's only one side of the story. The people who designed these programmes understood that if they wanted them to accomplish their stated goals – to empower people with mental health problems through supported employment on a large scale, they had to make them highly attractive from a business perspective, not just a humanitarian one.

Chapter 6
Bringing the Co-Production Model of Recovery Into the Mainstream

We forget about ourselves for a moment when we're helping someone else. Lending a hand could improve your self-esteem. There's a chance that whatever your diagnosis is, their's just might be worse. From the homeless to the privileged, mental illness affects us all, and with it comes the stigma we are beholden to combat. It's time to cash that reality check and make an investment in the future of mental wellness. Our lives will be the richer for it.
– Henry Boy Jenkins

This book is the fruit of the confluence between my own journey of recovery from mental ill health, and what I believe to be a time of significant transformation in the way that communities engage with their citizens who struggle with mental health problems. I have been preparing to write this for many years on a personal level, as an active Clubhouse member, writer, and aspiring speaker. However, in just the past five years a truly remarkable series of changes have transpired that have transformed the way Mosaic Clubhouse serves its members, including myself. I will explore this series of events in depth in this chapter, because I believe that it represents an extremely promising model of how communities around the world can take excellent care of their residents' mental health in the 21st century and beyond.

The transformation I'm referring to arose in response to our local mental health office's recognition of the success and efficiency of Mosaic Clubhouse's co-produced recovery programmes. The phrase 'co-production' simply refers to the way in which Clubhouse members are responsible for most of the tasks required to run their Clubhouse. In general terms, it can be defined as a collaborative approach in which everyone's skills, experience and knowledge are leveraged to achieve better outcomes and more efficient services. While Clubhouse International is not the only provider of co-produced recovery services, it is one of the more established organisations currently delivering such programmes on a global scale.

In addition to the empowering effects of co-production for members in recovery from mental ill health, this approach also keeps the costs associated with running a Clubhouse community remarkably low. After Mosaic Clubhouse's nearly two decades of operation as a joint project of the Borough of Lambeth and NHS Lambeth (we celebrated 20 years in 2014), these local agencies decided that they wanted to join forces with us at a larger scale, as part of a sweeping initiative called the Lambeth Living Well Partnership. While philosophical differences made these efforts a bit bumpy initially, the final result has surpassed everyone's expectations in its seamless integration of a more mainstream approach to community-based mental health care with a co-produced Clubhouse model. The Mosaic community takes great pride in providing one of the first such models in the world, and I'm hopeful that what we've accomplished will inspire imitation across the globe.

A Case Study of Mosaic Clubhouse as a Hybrid Approach to Co-Produced Recovery

The changes to Mosaic Clubhouse's operations that have taken place over the past five years have represented a synthesis that few would have believed possible previously. In a case study that she wrote for the Birmingham-based charitable organisation Governance International, Mosaic chief executive Maresa Ness outlines the process of negotiation that resulted in our Clubhouse's current incarnation here in Lambeth. I believe that this case study represents an invaluable resource for communities worldwide, and I will refer to it repeatedly throughout this chapter. The document is entitled Outcomes-Based Commissioning and Public Service Transformation in Mosaic Clubhouse, Lambeth, and the full text can be accessed on the Governance International website at www.govint.org.

Below is Ms. Ness's description of how it all started:

In 2010 the business model of Mosaic Clubhouse was challenged when a contract with the London Borough of Lambeth came to an end, and the local council asked the Clubhouse to expand its services to the 100 clients of a day-care centre for people with mental health issues. The new service contract was to be based on an outcomes framework. The main outcomes to be achieved included:

• Clients leading more productive lives by sharing their talents with a vibrant, inclusive community, resulting in stronger social networks, better mental health and improved skills;

• Increased take-up of education and employment opportunities;

- Increased self-confidence to make informed choices about their future.

The expectation was that people could be fast tracked through the system in 12 weeks by identifying their own recovery goals, and could be supported to meet them quickly. The Clubhouse was also asked to run an information service in partnership with Lambeth Mind for anyone in the borough with any queries, and to form partnerships with other organisations who would use the building on a sessional basis to enable people to be seen rapidly for talking therapies, housing advice etc.

As you'll know by now, one of the key features that define a Clubhouse community is that clinicians do not staff it, and therapeutic practices do not take place within its walls. This isn't just a loose guideline; it's a core principle that's at the heart of Clubhouse International's commitment to co-produced recovery. It's one of the thirty-six recovery standards that must be met by individual Clubhouses in order to receive certification from Clubhouse International. For Mosaic Clubhouse to be asked to deviate from this standard represented a threat not only to its programmatic integrity, but to its status as one of only ten international Clubhouse training centres, a privilege that requires re-certification every three years.

The expanded role that the Lambeth Council was asking Mosaic Clubhouse to fill also required the Clubhouse to move into a new building that would be more conducive to performing that role, and this added additional stress for the community at a time of uncertainty. However, the rest of Ms. Ness's case study outlines the almost miraculous way that the Mosaic Clubhouse community turned a major challenge to its identity into a stunning rebirth, by re-committing to the very co-production principles that the government's proposals had threatened to change:

There are 36 recovery and co-production standards that govern all Clubhouses, and they include standards such as "Membership is voluntary and without time limits." Performance against the 36 standards is assessed very closely by the international Clubhouse faculty, and includes a lengthy self-assessment and a three-day visit by a faculty staff and a faculty member. This then gives a "licence to operate" for between 1 - 3 years, depending on adherence to the standards.

As Mosaic Clubhouse is one of only 10 international training bases, it must always achieve 3 years accreditation. In the case of standard number 1 (above) commissioners were pressing for a "reablement" model, suggesting that it should be possible to offer anyone with a serious mental health condition an individualised twelve week programme that would enable them to set and achieve their recovery goals. This was not envisaged as being part of a Clubhouse programme, but as a separate 1:1 support. Standard 9 states "Clubhouse staff are sufficient to engage the membership, yet few enough to make carrying out their responsibilities impossible without member involvement."

Standard 10 states "Clubhouse staff have generalist roles. All staff share employment, housing, evening and weekend, holiday and unit responsibilities. Clubhouse staff do not divide their time between Clubhouse and other major work responsibilities that conflict with the unique nature of member / staff relationships."

Standard 13 states "The Clubhouse is located in its own physical space. It is separate from any mental health centre and is impermeable to other programmes."

These standards (and others) were at risk of being compromised by our new role as hosts of the Lambeth Living Well Partnership, which required the Clubhouse to offer space to other agencies; to deliver a 1:1 twelve-week programme to individuals; and to run an information service open to the public five days a week as a drop-in, e-mail or telephone service (the so-called information hub). It was also expected to open an enlarged café to the public so that people could "drop in" for information, food, and drink, and so that mental health professionals could use the café to meet their patients in a community setting. Finally, it was informed that the space identified for its education and employment department would be available for any other mental health organisations in the borough for use either for meetings, or running traditional drop-in activities, all of which fundamentally seemed to threaten the Clubhouse Model in the worst possible way.

However, the Clubhouse managed to agree on a wider co-produced service model, which meant that the Clubhouse involved members in the design and delivery of the new services. As a result, Mosaic Clubhouse agreed to deliver the information service "side by side," and to integrate the new 12-week offering into the regular Clubhouse work.

Clubhouse members were also heavily involved in the discussions at all times when a £1million refurbishment was planned on an existing council (ex-day centre) building. The building was adapted to meet the needs of a 21st century Clubhouse. It is light and airy with open spaces in all departments to support members to see the work being done each day, thereby encouraging engagement and a recovery journey.

The move on 30th April 2013 gave staff and members time to work together to fully equip the new building, plant the garden, review all policies and procedures, carry out all necessary training (in particular, health and safety and food hygiene as the café and information hub are both open to the public). The expanded service meant recruiting six extra staff and ensuring that all staff and more members were trained in the Clubhouse Model. The information hub formally opened in September 2013 while the Clubhouse component was operational immediately.

All aspects of the new service offered are co-delivered by staff and members. This means that there are even more opportunities for members, such as organising and hosting external agencies meetings; which includes laying out the room, meeting and greeting, signing in, giving directions, providing IT support, supplying food and refreshments, cleaning up, producing leaflets for the information hub, taking calls, face to face enquiries, presentations to other agencies etc. The Clubhouse now offers peer support in the community (as always) and externally to people in the information hub.

The potential threat originally posed by this significant change has instead become a really positive outcome for all concerned, and built an even stronger Clubhouse...

As you know, my focus in this book is on the benefits of Clubhouse International's Transitional Employment Programs for businesses, as well as for Clubhouse members. Mosaic Clubhouse's expanded role has made it possible for members to train in an even more diverse range of skill sets than was available to them previously, as part of their daily Clubhouse activity. Read over that list of tasks again: could your company use a ready-made, entry-level workforce that comes with guaranteed backup for absences? If so, it's in your interest to encourage your local government to support the expansion and integration of its mainstream community-based efforts with your local Clubhouse's programmes.

The recent transformation of Mosaic Clubhouse into a community hub for Lambeth residents with mental health problems has shown that applying the Clubhouse co-production model of recovery in a more mainstream context can yield extraordinary results for members and the community alike. I am proud to have participated in this historic transformation, and I hope to see many more like it emerge in the years to come, as part of a revolution in the way the world handles mental health care. If what you've read inspires you, I hope you will consider how your business might partner with your local Clubhouse to become part of the solution. The possibilities are truly endless.

Chapter 7
We Choose to Live With Dignity and Purpose

I am a deep believer in the power of the Fountain House model. To have a stigma-free, member-run, collegial sanctuary where you are taught the skills that can lead to a life where work and independent living are a possibility...not only engenders life-affirming hope, but, indeed, changes and saves lives.
– Glenn Close, Actress and Founder
of the American anti-stigma campaign
Bring Change 2 Mind

Thus far, this book has relied a great deal on formal research and the authority of non-members to convey the benefits of Clubhouse participation for people in recovery from mental ill health. I've taken this approach because I know that leaders in the world of business expect assertions of value to be fully backed up by concrete figures, and I have sought to establish that the Clubhouse model has been thoroughly validated in this way.

That said, however, I believe that ultimately it is Clubhouse members who are the true experts on their own journeys of recovery within Clubhouse communities. They are the ones who can tell us exactly how this model can help a wide variety of people to rebuild a sense of dignity, purpose, and self-esteem. Most of all, the stories of Clubhouse members serve to put a human face on recovery from mental ill health, and this is crucial to breaking the bonds of stigma that too often still serve to keep people with mental health problems socially isolated and underemployed.

The end of stigma begins with social contact between people who struggle with mental health problems and those who do not, and the experiences of shared productivity that comes with working side-by-side adds valuable fuel to that fire. This is why Clubhouse Transitional Employment Programs are vital not only to individual recovery, but to the struggle to end the stigma that still surrounds the subject of mental illness. Through the experience of interacting with TEP participants, other employees in a company can begin to view those with mental health problems as fellow humans who wish to feel a sense of belonging and contribution to society, and are as determined as anyone to earn that right. Participants in TEPs gain valuable skills and a sense of empowerment, and their co-workers gain a new view of mental illness not as a choice, but as a disease from which people can recover just as they do from any purely physical affliction.

Now that you've seen some of the facts and figures in support of the Clubhouse model in general, and TEPs in particular, it's time to hear the message from the lips of Clubhouse members themselves. In the remainder of this chapter, I will share a series of testimonials that provide an inspiring glimpse into how individuals from a variety of backgrounds have benefited from Clubhouse programmes, including TEPs. Their words offer compelling evidence that the human spirit can rebound from incredible challenges when nourished with love, empowerment, and positive expectation. I hope you enjoy reading these as much as I enjoyed compiling them.

Stories from Mosaic Clubhouse: Renewing Hope One Day at a Time

The testimonial below is actually a transcription from a video on the Mosaic Clubhouse website, in which my fellow member Coretta describes how participating in a TEP helped her begin to get inspired and excited about her future in a way she hasn't been for a long time. Her courageous efforts to re-enter the world of employment after a long absence speaks to the deep desire of many unemployed people with mental health problems to return to productive work:

Life before Mosaic was full of anxiety and stress, because I didn't have anywhere to go, I didn't have any friends. After I was diagnosed with schizophrenia I was sitting at home, having nothing to do, but I finally made an appointment to see a social worker who introduced me to Mosaic Clubhouse, and that was the start of my life…I was made to feel welcome, which is what I like about it. It's why I continue to come, because I met people who I didn't know and I was given work to do on my first day, which I didn't know how to do, but I was instructed by the members and staff, which I liked, because I was learning new things for the future…

Transitional Employment has changed my life drastically in a good way, because I didn't have any experience with office skills, but working at Mosaic really helped me in this field, because…I was actually trained there [in the Mosaic office] before I got this job. It was my first job in four years. Before my TEP, I had immigration issues because I didn't have the right to work in the UK, but after it came through Mosaic came forward and helped me to find this transitional employment, which was the start of my career.

After my TEP ended, the staff at Mosaic Clubhouse helped me a great deal to do a job search, and referred me to other agencies… I went for an interview which was good for me because I really really wanted to do work.

My aspiration for the future is to become a manager at a flagship store. I will always be a member of Mosaic Clubhouse no matter where I go, or how far I aspire.

As Coretta notes at the end of her testimonial, one of the central features of a Clubhouse community is that once they've become members, people are always welcome to participate in Clubhouse life, regardless of where their aspirations may take them. A good portion of TEP participants like Coretta go on to gain independent employment following their TEP, yet many of these people choose to remain connected to the community through events that are scheduled outside of their working hours. They say that it feels good to provide an example for new members of what is possible through Clubhouse participation, and to pass on the skills and knowledge they've learned to those just starting out on the path of recovery. It is a human need to feel needed, and while Clubhouses fulfil this need initially via their commitment to co-production, they continue to do so for members who have regained independence by continuing to welcome their participation for life, as colleagues and informal mentors for other members.

The following testimonial from a young man who wishes to be identified only by his initials, DM, is typical of many people who are surprised to find a resource like Mosaic Clubhouse available in their community:

When I came out of hospital and got better, I never thought there would be help for people who are stable but still trying to put things right. Until I looked for help and found Mosaic Clubhouse, I assumed there would only be help for people that are still in a severe mental condition.

For a long time I have been trying to get back on track and it has been a bumpy road with ups and downs. The peer support available at Mosaic Clubhouse sometimes helps just through speaking to someone who has the same day-to-day struggles as you, which means that you do not feel all alone.

Since coming to Mosaic Clubhouse, I have become more confident, learned new skills in gardening and also how to cook and work in a fully stocked kitchen.

I am now taking part in a TEP [Transitional Employment Program]: a temporary work position in a private hospital as a porter/food preparer. At first I was a bit nervous about the job but it went well. A support worker, Angela, was there to help me get settled in my placement, and I'll be supported by Mosaic Clubhouse throughout my placement which will last for nine months, after which another member of Mosaic Clubhouse will take over.

I am learning new cooking skills at work and also when contributing at the Clubhouse. And now I am using these skills and making more food for myself at home.

I hope to one day become a skilled full-time chef and I look forward to learning more.

DM's experience with the Clubhouse, and with his TEP in particular, has given him renewed hope for a sense of contribution and independence following recovery from mental illness. It illustrates the incredible power that returning to work has to support those with mental health problems in all aspects of their healing journey.

Another member, DP, speaks directly to the joy that many unemployed people with mental health problems feel upon being granted the opportunity to work again:

I have been unemployed for the past three years and miss being in full-time employment terribly. At Mosaic Clubhouse I was told about TEPs [Transitional Employment Programs] for members to attend, to gain work experience, up-to-date job references and the confidence to move ahead into independent employment. I myself have had a TEP arranged for me at Cambian Churchill Hospital in Kennington to work as a receptionist. This placement will enable me to provide good customer service and gain additional administrative skills.

Stories from The Meeting Place in San Diego: A Renewed Sense of Purpose and Confidence

The following two testimonials come from the Meeting Place Clubhouse in San Diego, California USA. This one is from Denise W., who was referred to the Clubhouse by a clinician who treated her for severe depression:

Ever since coming here in May, I've become part of a workforce team. I work in the kitchen, I help cook healthy organic lunches. I've almost lost 30 pounds since being here. The Clubhouse is great, members are great, staff are great, they're here to show support for everybody. They have resources that can help anybody that needs them. At this point, they've got me what they call a TE job, transitional employment. I'm very happy there, and I'm hoping that when my TEP job is up, that they will be keeping me there as a permanent employee. Before the Clubhouse, I had no purpose, and I'm glad I finally found it.

Tina had this to say about how her Clubhouse experience has helped her build more confidence:

One of the things that I appreciate the most working here at the Clubhouse and being a member is the team I work with, the staff and members. They have such a positive, uplifting feeling for me, and it makes me feel more confident. Some of the jobs [within the Clubhouse] I even found hard at first, but I was given a lot of encouragement, and I get to work on a team often, which I really like. I think that having more structure in my life has helped.

The handful of testimonials that I've been able to share in this chapter hardly begins to scratch the surface of the impact that Clubhouse TEPs have had on the lives of members around the world. By giving new members work to do from their first day, Clubhouses acknowledge that a sense of contribution is the best medicine to help people who have been out of work to rebuild their skills and independence. By providing a means for people to re-enter the workforce at a pace that works for them, Clubhouse TEPs are empowering people to regain a sense of productivity and a chance at greater self-reliance, within a framework of inter-dependence. This is truly the best-case scenario for people who have been disenfranchised due to mental ill health, whose greatest wish is to be given the opportunity to recover without judgment.

I hope that, as a forward-thinking business owner, you will consider the benefits that a partnership with your local Clubhouse's Transitional Employment Program might offer not only to the members you employ, but to your other employees and your bottom line as well. Like some of the members whose testimonies you've just read, you may be surprised to find in your local Clubhouse a hidden gem just waiting to be discovered.

Conclusion
Bringing a Message of Hope to the World

Whatever you can do, or believe you can, begin it. Boldness
has genius, power, and magic in it!
– Johann Wolfgang von Goethe

We've now reached the end of my little book, and I hope that it has inspired you to do your part to end stigma against people with mental health problems. I wish to thank you for reading this far, and for being prepared to take a stand for the empowerment of people like myself, whose deepest desire is to be seen as whole people with valuable contributions to make. Our greatest need is not for sympathy, but for opportunities to contribute and thereby achieve a renewed sense of hope and belonging. As a business owner, particularly if your business employs a number of people at the entry level, you are well-positioned to fulfil this need, and I hope you will take steps to do so in partnership with your local Clubhouse's Transitional Employment Program.

I recently had a very inspiring telephone conversation with a friend of mine named Jo, whom I met at an event focused on self-development. Jo shared with me how she is applying the knowledge she learned from this event to developing her public speaking skills. She asked me if I was interested in doing public speaking on mental health stigma and discrimination in the workplace, and I said 'yes.' I was somewhat surprised to find myself very excited by the idea of speaking in front of audiences.

Jo felt that my experience with mental health issues be valuable to share as a speaker, and she volunteered to be my accountability buddy to ensure that I practice my speaking skills regularly. Her belief in my potential as a speaker has been a tremendous boost to my self-confidence, and I wish to acknowledge her encouragement here.

I've been inspired to speak about my journey of recovery from mental ill health because of the positive response I've received when I've disclosed my history to my colleagues at Mosaic Clubhouse. They were amazed at what I had been through, and impressed with the way that I have come through it. One of them even remarked, "If you hadn't told us about your history, I would just have thought of you as an average guy, maybe struggling a bit with English because it is not your first language." This reminded me that not all reaction to my story from the general public will be negative, and that sharing can have a very positive and uplifting effect in the right context.

When I told my friends that I now plan to talk about my mental health experience on stage, they said, "Wow, good for you. You have a lot to tell. Your story will inspire many people and give them hope that true recovery from mental ill health is not just a dream, it is achievable. You are a living example." I would like to help more people like me, so they don't feel they are alone with their troubles. It is rewarding to feel that I am helping others, as it gives me a sense of the meaning behind my own journey.

In addition to the work I currently do to promote Mosaic Clubhouse, I aspire to spread the word about the power of Transitional Employment to revolutionise the way that people recover from severe mental health problems in communities around the world, through writing and public speaking in a variety of venues. If you would like to invite me to speak at your organisation or event, I can be reached at Mosaic Clubhouse, 65 Effra Road, London SW2 1BZ, England.

Once again, thank you for giving my book some of your time and attention. I look forward to joining forces in an effort to end stigma against mental health problems in the workplace and beyond.

Made in the USA
Charleston, SC
20 August 2016